INSOMNIA

NATURAL ALTERNATIVE STRATEGY.

SHEILA BER –
Naturopathic Consultant.

INTRODUCTION:

I'm a Microbiological/Chemical Technologist, who is currently working as a Naturopathic Consultant.

I'm writing this book to provide advice and help, to treat insomnia problems, by removing the root causes, rather than addressing the symptom only.

There are many internal and external factors, influencing the body and affecting how you feel, think, act, eat. These are all manifested in your sleep.

Much of the advice provided in this book, is from my microbiological/chemical background, as well as from my own personal experience.

I dedicate the book to both my dear sons: Phillip and Bernard.

The book is also dedicated to all who seek help,

to better their lives and to examine, at a fundamental level all the contributing factors to their health problems, that consequently lead to their insomnia problems.

*   *   *

INDEX:

What is insomnia?

Insomnia is a sleep disorder consisting of the inability to fall asleep easily, or stay asleep throughout the night. The frequency of persistent insomnia is high. Difficulty in initiating or maintaining refreshing restorative sleep.

Insomnia may cause dramatic impairments of psycho-social functions as well as on general quality of life.

It is the most common sleep disorder in our modern fast paced, industrial and technological world.

Insomnia affects <u>modestly</u> up to 50% of the adult population, and over 10% it is affecting the general population in a <u>chronic</u> form.

The basic causes contributing to insomnia are attributed to PSYCHOLOGICAL (EMOTIONAL), PSYCHIATRIC, and PHYSIOLOGICAL factors.

The impact of insomnia.

A person with insomnia can be experiencing one or more of the following:

Impaired daily functioning, Tiredness, inability to focus at work or at school, poor memory.

Slowed reaction time, and drowsiness, that may lead to accidents, headaches and body aches, obesity problems, inability to enjoy interpersonal relationships.

People with insomnia report poorer physical and mental well being, which includes sometimes higher levels of depression and anxiety.

Chronic insomnia occurring frequently, for over a month, is quite common in mood disorders such as Bipolar disorder, or major depression.

Depressive episodes are symptoms often causing sleep difficulties.

People having manic or hypo-manic episodes often find that they need less sleep than normal. If they get restful sleep, it is then not considered insomnia.

However, sleep disruption or insomnia can trigger a mania state in people who have mood disorders.

Some medications used in the treatment of bipolar disorder can cause difficulty sleeping, including the following anti depressants:

Cymbalta (Duloxetine)
Effexor   (Venlafaxine)
Lexapro   (Escitalopram)
Paxil   (Paroxetine)
Prozac   (Fluxetine)

Assessment and causes of insomnia.

1. Nervous system: The nervous system acts as a thermometer, as it is linked to all psychological and physiological aspects of the body, it is very sensitive to any changes or disruptions to the other systems in your body. Its sensitivity is manifested into the body and brain sleeping state.

**Negative emotions**: anxiety, anger, fears, worries, obsessions.
All of these emotions interfere with a good night sleep.

**Solutions**: 1) **For anxiety & nervousness**: **Passion flower**
extract – Take 10-15 drops in ¼ cup of water, for about 3
weeks. Pause for 1 week, and if symptom continue,
repeat the above, and stop when feeling calmer.

1) **Holy Basil** – 1-3x a day, and you take 1 during the night
if awake.
The herb strengthens the immune system, and produces
body calmness.
2) **Dong Quai** – 1-3x a day, and take 1 during night if
cannot sleep.
This herb is known as Angelica. It balances hormones, and
provides tranquilizing effect on the body and the mind.

3) **B6 & B-Complex** - 50-100 mg. - take 2- 3x a day. B-6 is
more effective if taken with other B vitamins, along with
vitamin C 500-1000 mg. This vitamin relaxes all muscles
including heart and lungs. It lowers the production of the
stress hormone Cortisol.

It functions as a coenzyme in more than one hundred metabolic processes. It is required for normal brain function, and for the nervous system. It also boosts immunity.

5) <u>Calcium & Magnesium</u> - 1000-1200 mg Calcium & 500-600 mg. Magnesium, divided in 2 - twice a day. It is a natural relaxant combination, which has a calming effect on the nervous system. (soda can actually strip away calcium).

6) <u>Magnesium Citrate/Malate</u> – 500-1000 mg. Take only if you feel very restless, or experience Restless leg syndrome.

<u>Note</u>: This Magnesium form should be taken separately and in addition to Calcium &Magnesium supplement. Again, only when experiencing restlessness and anxiety. It relaxes muscles including heart and lungs, provides natural calm, reduces stress and insomnia, helps maintain low blood pressure, promotes healthy cell production, and promotes healthy pH balance.

In extreme nervousness state: take <u>Valerian extract</u> - 5-10 drops on your tongue, swash, and swallow, <u>for immediate relief</u> within about 2 minutes!

<u>Note</u>: <u>Take Valerian extract occasionally, ONLY when in extreme stress and anxiety. Discontinue when symptoms subside.</u>

<u>2. Circadian rhythm sleep disorder (CR)</u>: If rhythm is disrupted due to travel, nightly shift work, irregular and late bedtime, the body produces less Melatonin(sleep inducer), and more of Cortisol (stress hormone). The correct ratio is to have the body produce more Melatonin, and less Cortisol.

<u>Solutions</u>: 1) To get adequate amount of Melatonin, you need to expose your body to sunlight during the day. <u>In the winter</u>, you can supplement sunlight, by using special WHITE LIGHT SYSTEM, usually used for Seasonal Affective Disorder (SAD). It works! Try it!

2) Take _Melatonin_ supplement – 1 capsule/tablet 3-6 mg. 15 minutes before bedtime.

3) _To reduce high Cortisol level_, usually associated with anxiety, take _Colustrum_ 500 mg 1-3 capsules a day.

4) _Pantothenic acid (B5)_ 100-250 mg. once a day.

It can also be taken during the night if you are unable to fall asleep, or remain asleep. It is called the STRESS B-vitamin.

If you take one or all of the supplements listed above, under _Nervous system_, your _Cortisol_ hormone level should remain low. You will lower your anxiety level and feel more calm.

3. Digestive system: Indigestion causes body unrest, as it requires much oxygen to aid digestion, depriving other parts of the body from getting adequate oxygen supply to function well and feel restful.

Solutions: 1) Take _digestive enzymes_ that contain _Ox bile_ and _HCl_ (Hydrochloric acid).

A good brand is "Now" called: SUPER ENZYMES, can be obtained at any health store.

2) <u>Your last meal</u> should be approximately 3 hours before bedtime.

<u>4. Hormonal imbalance</u>: *Hormonal imbalance can disrupt overall body functions, leading to poor sleep patterns.*

<u>Solutions</u>: *1) Take a <u>periodical blood test</u>. If imbalance present, address it with your medical practitioner.*

2) <u>Dong Quai</u> – Take 500 mg. 1-3 capsules a day, for 2 weeks.

Dong Quai is also used for effectively treating PMS, arthritis, and lowering blood pressure. It has a calming effect.

It promotes hormonal balance, in men and women.

3) <u>Wild yam</u> – 1 capsule 2-3 per day, for 2 weeks.

<u>5. Thyroid imbalance</u>: *Check your Thyroid level. Imbalance disrupts overall body functions.*

Solutions: Take a periodical blood test. If imbalanced, address it with your medical practitioner.

6. High blood pressure: *If your blood pressure is high, address it with your medical doctor.*

The following natural herbs can promote and maintain low blood pressure.

Solutions:

1) Turmeric: ¼ teaspoon in ½ cup boiled water. Cool and drink 2-3 times a day. It is a blood thinner, anti inflammatory, and also promotes lower blood pressure.

2) Celery: Eat 2-3 sticks daily. It works!

3) Magnesium Citrate/Malate: It relaxes all muscles, organs including the heart.

It relaxes also the venal and arterial system, by expanding them, and allowing blood to flow through, without excessive pressure.

4) *Keep your <u>Sodium</u> intake <u>low.</u>*

5) *Take <u>Potassium - 99 mg</u>. 1-2 capsules daily. It will reduce your blood pressure. It will also keep your electrolyte fluids balanced, as well as balanced blood pH.*

<u>7. pH imbalance:</u> *Our body is usually more acidic, and therefore pH imbalanced.*

This is due to our modern diet that is highly acidic, plus higher stress level, resulting in higher microbial level in our body. Higher microbial level results in a higher level of inflammation.

Microbes produce acid through their metabolism.
Acidic body is a restless body, and deprived of Oxygen.

Alkalizing is necessary, because it will reduce microbial level, and will promote higher oxygen level. It will also produce general calmness, which is helpful to induce better sleep experience.

6) Keep your <u>Sodium</u> intake <u>low.</u>

<u>Solutions</u>:

1) Keep the intake of the following, to a <u>minimum</u>: <u>sugar, carbohydrates, white flour products, coffee, cocoa,</u> <u>Coca-Cola, beer, red meat, wheat, barley, oils (that are low in omega), fats, pickled foods containing vinegar.</u>

<u>Note</u>: Other important food items are also acidic, but they are essential to our daily diet, and cannot be avoided.

To neutralize body acidity (acid pH), I recommend a simple and a very effective remedy, as following:

*Take <u>**Baking Soda**</u> (Sodium Bi-Carbonate) - ½ teaspoon in 1 cup water, stir well, and drink. Take it after a heavy meal, to also aid digestion. It provides quick relief for indigestion, as well as providing you with more energy.*

It balances your body pH, and it discourages the growth of unfriendly micro-organism (gram negative bacteria).

8. High microbial level (including Viruses, Bacteria, Fungus, Yeast, Worms:

A healthy body generally hosts friendly as well as unfriendly bacteria, including yeast, at an acceptable level and in balance.

Friendly bacteria are called: <u>Aerobic</u> bacteria.
Unfriendly bacteria are called <u>Anaerobic</u> bacteria.
Anaerobic bacteria function without oxygen, and if in excessive number, and out of balance in the intestinal flora, it will contribute to the development of infection and inflammation in the body.

Yeast and Fungus, also, if at an excessive level, the result is an unbalanced intestinal flora. They are another major contributing factor to body infections and inflammation.

What causes imbalance in our intestinal flora?

Answer: *Highly acidic diet, high stress level, hormonal imbalance, high sugar and carbohydrates intake, high alcohol intake, food toxins including bacteria, yeast, fungus, worms, and viruses, and environmental toxins.*

Solutions: *1) Take <u>probiotics</u> containing 5-10 billions active cells of <u>Acidophilus and Bifidus</u> (friendly bacteria) 1-2 capsules a day, with a glass of <u>warm water</u>, to activate them.*

1) <u>Alkalize</u>: Neutralize your body acidic pH.

Acidic pH contributes to a higher presence of microbes, and microbes metabolites release even more acid into our body tissues. It is like a vicious circle.

9. Vitamin D3 deficiency:

Vitamin D is now recognized as a major player in contributing to overall human health. It improves sleep patterns. It improves your mind and your health in general.

Research has shown the links between vitamin D and a strong immune system, healthy heart and strong mind. All of these things are also helped by better sleep achieved when the body gets an adequate supply of vitamin D3.
The D3 form is the most readily absorbed by the human body.

Recommended intake: 3,000 I.U. - 7,000 I.U daily. Best taken with Omega oil, for maximum absorption. It is fat soluble.

10. Alcohol and coffee : Minimize your alcohol
and coffee intake. They can interfere with REM sleep.

Do not consume them after 2 pm, as they will also cause
interrupted sleep patterns.

11. General pain & muscle pain:

*Pain triggers poor sleep. The major causes of sleep loss due to
pain are back pain, headaches, abdominal pain, and facial
pain. Also, musculoskeletal pain, which includes Arthritis and
Fibromyalgia, can lead to poor sleep. Pain from cancer, the
disease itself and its treatment, is also a major offender
causing poor sleep. Pain is a serious intrusion to sleep.*

*Here are tips to obtain better sleep, for anyone suffering
from chronic pain:*

- Limit caffeine consumption, and consume before 2 pm.

- Limit alcohol intake.

- Avoid vigorous exercise. However, light exercise in the afternoon can be helpful.

- Take a brief nap in the afternoon, no more than 20 minutes.

The use of pain killers and/or sleeping pills can be effective, however only under the supervision of a physician.

- Practice relaxation exercises, such as deep abdominal breathing.

- Aim for a regular bedtime.

- Create a calm environment.

- Keep your bedroom completely dark. Keep temperature at an ideal slightly cool range: 18-20 degrees Celsius. It helps you breathe and sleep better.

- Keep you room humidified in the winter. Dry air can make sleep difficult. Invest in high quality steam humidifier. Alternatively, you may place a plastic bowl filled with water, beside your bed. It is simple and very effective!

12. Restless leg syndrome:

Restless legs syndrome (RLS) is a neurological disorder characterized by throbbing, pulling, creeping, or other unpleasant sensations in the legs and an uncontrollable, sometimes, overwhelming urge to move them. Symptoms occur primarily at night when a person is relaxing or at rest and can increase in severity during the night.

Moving the legs relieves the discomfort. The sensations range in severity from uncomfortable to irritating to painful.

The most distinctive or unusual aspect of the condition is that lying down and trying to relax activates the symptoms. Most people with RLS have difficulty falling asleep and/or staying asleep. If left untreated, the condition causes exhaustion and daytime fatigue.

Symptoms are partially or totally relieved by movement such as walking or stretching.

Causes are many and some of them are: smoking, alcohol consumption, iron deficiency (Anemia), anxiety, B vitamins and mineral deficiency

Natural treatment recommended for RLS:

a. Reduction and or <u>elimination of alcohol, nicotine</u>, and <u>caffeine</u> from diet can be very helpful.

b. <u>Moderate exercise</u> helps the condition.

c. <u>Iron</u> tablets taken in <u>vegetable form</u>, can be very helpful.

d. <u>Magnesium Citrate</u> – 500-800 mg – two (2) x a day. This mineral is extremely helpful, due to its muscle relaxant effect. It helps lower your blood pressure, and keeps your nervous system in optimum health.

e. *Vitamin B6* – *100mg- 1-2 times a day.*

f. *Folic acid* – *1-5 mg – once a day. It is extremely beneficial for all neurological disorders, including restlessness.*

g. *Massage* - *A natural way to treat restless leg syndrome. Massaging or kneading your calf muscles helps promote blood flow to the area, therefore helping to relieve restless legs.*

13. Electromagnetic radiation and sensitivity:

Increasing numbers of people are beginning to suspect or believe that exposure to EMF (Electromagnetic field) generated by electrical devices lead to a host of health problems. Some of the health problems blamed on EMF exposure include: Insomnia, Headaches, and the following:

- *Mental fog*
- *Vague fatigue*

- *Cancers like Leukemia*
- *Hair loss*
- *Immune system weakness*
- *Skin problems*
- *Depression*
- *Digestive problems*
- *Anxiety and restlessness.*

A study has found that heavy exposure to mobile phones shortened stage 3 and 4 sleep as well as REM latency.

The most important thing to do to avoid EMF side effects is to shield the home or at least the body. There is now an official designation of EMF sensitivity on the medical code books.

Natural treatment recommended for protection:

- *Limit your cell phone usage prior to sleep*
- *Keep your cell phone at a suitable distance from your body while sleeping*
- *Take iodine supplements regularly*
- *Try using a cell phone with a relatively lower SAR level.*
- *Minimize your usage of your computer or laptop – if possible.*
- *Wearing or using scalar pendants or shields (considered an unproven method) which are claimed by proponents to afford some protection. One of them is called Q-Link. Personally, I find Q-Link extremely helpful.*
- *Remove the alarm clock from your night table, and place it at reasonable distance of approximately 6 feet away. Cover it at night, to allow total darkness in the room.*
- *Wear a neodymium magnet disk, North Pole (negative) side on the skin. See instructions below.*

**Place <u>magnet`s north pole</u> (negative) <u>side down</u>, facing the skin, of your tummy area, the center of the body.

Many people are practicing the use of magnets just before going to sleep. They can be worn also during the day.

The North Pole side of the magnet is very soothing, relaxing, and has magical health benefits. It is healing, as well as promoting better sleep.

To hold the magnet in place, place a dime on top of the night wear, just over the magnet. The dime will stick to the magnet, holding it in place.

You can remove the magnet as soon as you get up in the morning.

Do the above nightly, to promote a calm sleep.

**It is important that you make sure that you <u>only</u> place the <u>NORTH (negative) side on your body</u>. The South side excites the body and has the opposite effect.

To many people, this magnet works like a charm, as it relaxes and provides them with a restful sleep every night. It works! Try it, you have got nothing to lose!

The rare earth neodymium magnets are among the most powerful rare earth magnets. In the health industry, they are very popular. In the alternative health field, the neodymium magnet is used to cure many disorders including muscle pain.

According to health scientists, the neodymium magnets are believed to have the ability to reduce injury recovery time and inflammation. Apart from that, it is also capable of enhancing normal health by stimulating blood circulation.

Using magnets for health is very beneficial because they are free of harmful side effects, and non invasive at the same time. Magnets provide you with energy! They are an important source of energy.

The magnetic instruments used to deliver health benefits include jewellery and massage paraphernalia.

Magnetic bracelets and other magnetic jewellery are generally used to relieve pains in the muscles and joints. Even in the post-operative period, the rare earth magnets can be of great help. It relieves the pain.
*It also promotes a good sleep pattern.

Electrochemistry provides many interesting theories that support the medical applications of magnets.

By using magnetism, the health benefits you could enjoy include reduction in stress, relief from insomnia and migraine. Studies have shown that with prolonged use, you can have long term health, such as more energy and vitality. If you suffer from migraine, wearing a magnetic necklace can help relieve headaches and reduce the severity. Unlike painkillers, health magnets do not block the pain signal to your brain.

They work directly on the area of pain. *This is the reason why neodymium and other health magnets should be placed as close to the point of pain as possible. Other ailments gain relief with rare earth magnets are chronic pain, muscles stiffness and arthritic pain.*

The static magnetic fields, produced by wearing magnets for health, can reduce the inflammation by penetrating through the skin, and deep into the tissues, and deeper into the blood streams.

The negative magnetic field (North Pole side) produces negative ions, which are responsible for normalizing the metabolic functions and assisting in reducing painful condition triggered by inflammation or cell degeneration.

Once the negative magnetic field has made contact with your skin, the damaged cells will react with it causing realignment of ions into their respective and proper position.

Eventually, the damaging of cells will stop and the healing will start over several days.

The magnetic fields produced by the permanent magnets <u>*enhance and regulate your blood circulation*</u> *with their interaction with the iron content in the blood. The magnetism goes deep into the skin and attracts the iron in the blood, stirring movement in the blood stream.*

*   * To get further information on healing Neodymium magnets, go to:*

http://www.sooperarticles.com/health-fitness-articles/general-health-articles/what-rare-earth-magnets-do-health-68471.html

14. Noise : *There are many people losing sleep due to external and internal noise in their environment.*

Experts say the intensity, abruptness, regularity, intrusiveness, familiarity and regularity of noises all affect sleep.

Noise at levels as low as 40 decibel, or as high as 70 decibels generally keep us awake. However, the absence of a familiar noise can also disrupt sleep. City dwellers may have trouble falling asleep without the familiar sounds of traffic. Or a traveler may find it difficult to sleep without the familiar tick, tick, tick of the alarm clock at home.

Some noise, although annoying at first, can gradually be ignored, allowing sleep to follow. However, important noise, like a parent's baby crying, a smoke alarm or even one's own name being called, are not easily assimilated and generally snap us awake.

Solutions:
1. White noise machine – "Sleepmate"

To understand the promise of white noise, one must first understand its mechanics. In its purest form, it is not really noise at all.

White noise, which is also known as white sound, is a combination of sound frequencies in equal amounts. Just like a white beam of light is made up of all the colors in the color spectrum, white noise is made up of all the sound frequencies.

Because it incorporates all sound frequencies from high sounds to very low sounds, it has a very beneficial noise cancelling or "masking" effect.

White noise sounds like a slow soothing "whoosh".

any say it is the sound of the rain, or the waves gently caressing the shore, or the wind blowing through the trees. It is a very peaceful sound that is instinctively soothing and calming to the ears and minds of humans of all ages. White noise is actually a sound given to us by Mother Nature, in the same way as she has provided us with water and air.

On the market there is the electro-mechanical sound conditioner called "Sleepmate".

The "Sleepmate" mechanically makes a "real" sound as opposed to a reproduced or simulated sound like other white noise machines.

It does not loop. By "looping", I mean the playing of a recorded or simulated segment of sound over and over. Most other white noise machines do loop but some hide it better than others.

Getting a machine that doesn't loop is really important. If you can detect a repetitive quality in the sound (such as a chirp that repeats over and over every 5 seconds), then that can be as annoying as the sound you are trying to mask.

2. Background soothing music:

Play calm, peaceful music such as the sound of ocean waves, water drops, or gentle wind blowing.
3. Ear plugs: *Many find them also, to be quite helpful.*

4. Acoustic insulation of the walls and the ceiling:

Consult with an acoustic contractor, or with an engineer. Sometimes is it extremely worthwhile to invest in such insulation, in order to have a lasting peace of mind. The results are definitely worth all the efforts involved in such a project.

Inquire about insulation for: 1. <u>Low frequency noise</u> 2. <u>High frequency noise</u>, as well as 3. <u>Impact noise.</u>

<u>*Materials used*</u>*:*

<u>Quiet Rock drywall 5/8" 1-2 layers</u>, <u>green glue, furring HAT channel</u>, <u>mass loaded vinyl barrier sheets</u>, <u>ROXUL Safe & Sound 3". Ensure the covering of all studs with acoustic insulation tape,</u> which is extremely important, in noise reduction.

Collect all the necessary information, and address any or all of the above. Get quotes from several contractors, and ask them what their specific plan is, the material used, their fee, time frame for completing the project, <u>warranty</u>, and recommendations.

Have it all clear in writing with the contractor's signature. Remember to obtain an <u>official receipt</u> upon payment.

15. Temperature and its effect on your sleep:

The point at which sleep is disturbed due to temperature or climate conditions varies from person to person. Generally, temperatures above 75 degrees Fahrenheit (24 degrees Celsius) and below 54 degrees (12 degrees Celsius) will awaken people.

The optimum temperature suitable for comfortable sleep, is 18-20 degrees Celsius (64-68 degrees Fahrenheit).

16. Altitude:

The higher the altitude, the greater is the sleep disruption. Generally, sleep disturbance becomes greater at altitudes of 13,200 feet or more. The disturbance is thought to be caused by diminished oxygen levels and accompanying changes in respiration. Most people adjust to new altitudes in approximately two to three weeks.

17. Dust Mites:

1. Within 10 years, dead dust mites and their waste can double the weight of your <u>mattress.</u>

<u>Make sure to use Bed Bug and Dust Mites proof, pillow and mattress protector covers.</u> They are your first line of defence against dust allergies! They also keep the pillow and mattress cool, which helps to sleep better.

Purchase a good brand that will last you a lifetime.

There are several good brands, one of them is: SecureSleep™ Bed Bug Mattress Cover Sets - Block dust mites too - at Website:

<u>www.allergybuyersclub.com</u>.

They sell similar products at different price range.

2. <u>Change your pillowcase 2-3 times a week.</u> Your sleep quality will tremendously improve. You will notice the difference!

<u>18. Adequate Pillow and Mattress for optimum support:</u>

<u>a. Choose a firm Mattress.</u> You can support your back by choosing a firm mattress. Though it may take 1-2 weeks to adjust to, it's well worth the investment and will be of great help in the long run.

Mattresses that sink or are too soft, allow the spine to move too deeply into a curve. This may result in leaving you with a back ache.

b. Use a medium firm Pillow. It will provide your head and the neck better support. A rolled hand towel can be placed under your neck if necessary. A medium firm pillow may be also placed, under your knees, and lower legs for a more relaxed, natural position.

pH imbalance impacting your sleep. How to alkalize?

Why acidic pH contributes to a higher microbial level in our body?

Answer: Acidic pH is high in H (Hydrogen) ions, and low in O2 (oxygen) ions, thus enabling anaerobic bacteria and other harmful microbes to multiply and function without the presence of Oxygen. If they are at an excessive level, they cause harm to the body. They produce infections and inflammation.

How to alkalize?

The simplest method is as following: Take ½ teaspoon of baking soda (Sodium Bicarbonate) in 1 cup water. Stir well, and drink. With the drink please take 1 capsule of Potassium Citrate 99 mg. in order to balance body electrolytic fluid.

Sodium and Potassium have to be in balance for the body to function at an optimum level. That will also help keep blood pressure in balance, and the heart pumping at an optimal rate!

Baking soda drink increases your oxygen level, thus increasing energy. It helps in improving digestion.

Taking the Baking soda drink is especially beneficial, following a heavy meal.

If you feel that you are highly acidic, you may repeat the above procedure, twice during the day.

Breathing problems and treatment:

To breath at optimal level, the trachea air pipe should be clear of inflammation and phlegm.

The inflammation has to be addressed by either taking medication if severe, and/or by treating it with natural supplements as follows:

1. Cod liver oil – *2-4 Tbsp daily.*
2. Turmeric – *1/4 tsp in 1/2 boiling water. Cool and drink warm 3x a day, to get rid of the phlegm.*
3. Beta Carotene – *10,000 I.U. – 2x a day.*
4. Vitamin D3 – *3,000-5,000 I.U. daily.*
5. Honey – *1 tsp 3x a day, without water. Allow the honey to use its anti bacterial properties, without rinsing it down with water, for about 15 minutes.*

Your pulmonary airways will also feel expanded, allowing you to breathe much better!

6. <u>*Probiotics*</u> *– 5-10 Billion active cells, in capsules 1-2x a day. They help fight inflammation very effectively!*

<u>*To expand your pulmonary airways and lungs,*</u> *the following supplements are also strongly recommended:*

1. <u>*Magnesium Citrate/Malate*</u> *– 500 mg. 2-3x a day.*
2. <u>*Honey*</u> *- 1/2 – 1 tsp - 3x a day, without water.*
3. <u>*Cod liver oil (bottle)*</u> *– 2-4 Tablespoons a day.*
4. <u>*Black seeds (Kalonji seeds)*</u> *– 1/4 tsp chewed or crushed well. Swallow with 1/2 cup warm water, 2 times daily. The seeds can be purchases at any East Indian store at a reasonable price. It is guaranteed to well expand the airways!* <u>*Kalonji seed*</u> *is a wonder seed, and has been used to cure many illnesses, for thousands of years, in many countries, by many cultures.*

Try also Kalonji oil – 1 tsp with 1/4 cup warm water. It helps to get deep sleep, and it is very beneficial for the liver, pancreas, and other organs.

Biochemical levels and periodical blood tests:

Blood tests are very common.

When you have routine checkups, your doctor will recommend blood tests to see how your body is working.

The following should be checked every 6 or 12 months:

- Hemoglobin count,
- White blood cell count,
- ESR (indicates inflammation level),
- Iron level,
- B12 - vitamin level,

- *Vitamin A level,*
- *Cortisol level (indicates stress level),*
- *Potassium level,*
- *Allergy tests.*

Daily microbial and chemical toxins elimination, and how it will improve your sleep.

When your body is burdened with toxins, bodily functions are disturbed and therefore work inefficiently. As a result this will also affect the chemical reactions in the brain. Consequently your body will feel unrested, along with the inability to fall asleep, or maintain a good night sleep.

Chemical and microbial toxins include the following:

bacterial/yeast/fungal overgrowth
- chronic parasitic infection
- chronic viral infection
- mercury dental amalgams
- liver, kidney & intestinal problems
- sluggish lymph & skin elimination
- heavy metals
- pesticides & herbicides
- chronic use of pharmaceutical drugs
- food chemicals & additives
- food allergies & sensitivities
- refined sugar, refined flour
- hydrogenated and trans fats
- coffee, alcohol & tobacco
- anger & resentment
- chronic worry, fear & sadness.

Staying healthy involves the awareness of toxins, the avoidance and elimination of toxins, and the nutritional repair to the cellular damage created by these toxins in your body. There are many toxins you can definitely avoid. Become knowledgeable and choose wisely.

There are toxins that you are not able to avoid, and therefore detoxification programs are of paramount importance, where ingesting toxins from your food and water, inhaling toxins from the air, and absorbing toxins through your skin are a daily occurrence.

To become and remain healthy, eliminating and excreting the presence of these illness-producing substances from your body is not only useful, but also vital for experiencing wonderful health.

Performing a regular detoxification program in order to maintain great overall health is like daily brushing and flossing your teeth in order to maintain great dental health.

The main organs in your body for ridding yourself of these toxins, and eliminating waste products are: the bowels, the liver, the kidneys, the lymphatic circulation, the skin and the lungs.

Fantastic health involves keeping these organs and systems well tuned. Detoxification programs emphasize and assist these organs of elimination to excrete toxins and wastes effectively.

Toxin accumulation can also lead to the generation of free radicals. Free radicals are naturally occurring in the body, yet with the addition of toxins there is more generated, which overtime can be harmful. Free radicals are a highly reactive, extremely unstable chemical compounds, that cause tissue destruction by attacking protein, DNA and cell membranes. Excessive free radical damage leads to numerous degenerative conditions, advanced aging and even contributes to the development of cancer.

Toxin build-up leads to inflammation in the body. This in return causes the inflammatory response. Although inflammation can be protective for the body, chronic inflammation is rather destructive and leads to various degenerative conditions, including auto-immune diseases.

Treatment to promote efficient bowel elimination:

1. Eat foods high in Fibre:

Fibre rich foods such as fruits, vegetables and whole grains are essential in promoting good bowel elimination.

A high fibre diet makes stools softer to pass, thus creating less straining, less constipation and the possibility for haemorrhoids.

Daily dietary fibre is a natural remedy for many digestive problems.

You will notice a positive change in your bowel functions, with an increase of fibre in your diet. It's ideal to have 1-2 bowel movements a day.

Psyllium Husk Fibre - is another alternative. It can be taken 1-2x a day, 1 tbsp mixed in 1 cup water. It works like a charm. Psyllium Husk can be purchased at any Health Food store.

2. Daily exercise:

If you don't like to exercise, you can start by walking more, taking the stairs instead of the elevator, and doing water aerobics, such as swimming.

Bicycling or stationary cycling is a good way to go. It exercises also the abdominal muscles, which help in bowel regularity.

Adding abdominal crunches or sit ups, to your exercise routine is very helpful in preventing constipation and promoting good bowel elimination.

3. Drink 6-8 cups of water daily:

Water is very beneficial to optimal health, and also to promote good bowel elimination. Water is also a natural stool softener if we drink enough of it.

Maintaining the colon moist by drinking an adequate amount of water, makes it easier for bowel elimination, and also along with fibre, water helps to sweep toxins away from the bowel. This helps keep your digestive system as a whole healthy, so that it can function more efficiently.

Water can be consumed in the form of soup, juice, coffee, regular tea or herbal tea.

4. Take Probiotics: *1- 2x a day, with 1/2 cup warm water.*

They positively help clean the colon from unwanted microbes, including yeast and harmful bacteria. They promote healthy bowel movements. You'll notice the difference!

5. Nutrition:

Eating a whole foods diet can help decrease toxin exposure to the system.

Avoid processed foods which contain unnecessary toxins. Also, eating a diet which is more alkalizing in nature can help decrease acid production in the system, and decrease toxin load in the body.

6. Rest:

Relaxation and adequate sleep are essential for proper organ function which is necessary for adequate removal of toxins.

7. Elimination through the skin:

Bathe away body toxins by treating yourself to a bath containing Epsom salts, which contain magnesium that's deficient in many of us, and baking soda, which is a pH balancing agent.

Bathe in moderately hot water, for about 20 minutes. The toxins will be removed from your body, via the skin.

You can bathe in Epsom salt daily, or 2-3x a week.

It is best to use a natural loofa, a semi-soft fibrous sponge, to open up your pores by gently scrubbing the Epsom solution all over your body.

8. Talk to your Doctor:

Please talk to your Naturopathic Doctor about which personalized toxin elimination plan would be best for you. Laboratory tests can be run to determine exactly which toxin is burdening your system, followed by an individualized plan to aid elimination.

Children and insomnia:

Lack of sleep in children or sleep deprivation may lead to cognitive and physical problems. Children may for example, have difficulty concentrating in school. They may demonstrate behaviour patterns that are more aggressive than normal.

Children may also act irritated when they are deprived of sleep.

Some doctors recommend Melatonin treatment for children suffering from chronic insomnia. Because there are no guidelines for giving Melatonin to children, parents should be cautious about administering this supplement to their children.

Allowing children to stay up late on weekends will only contribute to accumulated sleep deprivation with time. Make sure you talk to your child about how important sleep is.

Lifestyle changes including limiting television viewing up to 4 hours before bed may be all that is necessary to help your child sleep. If you aren't sure what steps to take, talk with your child's paediatrician or health provider for more advice about curing insomnia in children.

Supplements for children - to help induce sleep:

- Passion flower Extract - 10-20 drops in ¼ cup water, just before bedtime. Take it for about 2 weeks and stop for 1 week.

Take only upon onset of anxiety and restlessness. Passion flower is considered a very safe herb.

- *Melatonin* – 3-5 mg. capsule/tablet, 15 minutes before bedtime.

- *Vitamin B5* –(Pantothenic acid) – The vitamin may help to manage stress from psychological strain, migraines, chronic fatigue syndrome, and smoking and alcohol cessation.

Pantothenic acid has long been known to be essential for consistent antibody production.

Take one tablet 25-50 mg. just before bedtime. You can take it in the middle of the might, if unable to stay asleep.

- *Vitamin B6* - (Pyridoxine) - Pyridoxine is an especially important vitamin for maintaining healthy nerve and muscle cells and it aids in the production of DNA and RNA, the body's genetic material. It is necessary for proper absorption of vitamin B12 and for the production of red blood cells and cells of the immune system.

Vitamin B6 is required for the production of Serotonin and helps to maintain healthy immune system functions.

Vitamin B6 is indicated for the treatment of anemia, neurologic disturbances, seborrhoeic dermatitis, and cheilosis. In combination with <u>folic acid</u> and <u>vitamin B12</u>, vitamin B6 lowers homocysteine levels which is an amino acid linked to heart disease and stroke, and possibly other diseases.
<u>*Take one 25 mg. tablet before bedtime*</u>*. You can take it in the middle of the might, if unable to stay asleep.*

- <u>Lecithin</u> – Give your child a warm glass of milk before bed. Add to the milk 1 tablespoon of <u>Lecithin</u> granules, and 1 tsp <u>honey</u>. Lecithin induces sleep and also promotes a healthy nervous system.

- <u>L-Theanine</u> - (An amino acid extracted from tea leaves) – 1 capsule before bedtime. It reduces anxiety and promotes calm.

- <u>Light snack before bedtime</u> a light snack approximately two hours before bedtime, as falling and staying asleep can be difficult if the child is hungry.

A healthy snack can help take the edge off of hunger and helps him/her sleep through the night.

The snack should contain mostly carbohydrates and a small amount of protein.

This combination may help increase the availability of Tryptophan (an amino acid that helps induce sleep) to the brain. It will also help increase Serotonin level.

A few pre-bedtime snack ideas include:

- *A warm glass of milk with honey,*
- *A small bowl of oatmeal*
- *Cereal with low-fat milk*

- *Yogurt with granola sprinkled on top*
- *Half of a bagel topped with peanut butter*
- *Five whole-grain crackers with one ounce cheese*
- *Sliced apple with one ounce cheese or peanut butter.*
- *A banana.*

Good night!
pleasant dreams my friend!

Sheila Ber, 2015.

Disclaimer,

Sheila Ber BIOGRAPHY   2015.

Professionally:

I'm a **Microbiological/Chemical Technologist**, currently working as a **Naturopathic consultant**.

I worked in the fields of Microbiology and Chemistry, for about 15 years, in the Pharmaceutical as well as the Cosmetics industries.

I was also involved in Research & Development, and in formulations of a large variety of products.

Personally:

In general, I'm an unconventional person, though over the years, I have become a bit more conventional.
I like things to be straight, simple, and uncomplicated.

I enjoy helping people, and giving advice
 wherever, and whenever I can.

I view all things, situations, from different perspectives, and refrain from passing judgment on anyone.

We are who we are, because of the countless of reasons and circumstances that made us who we are and where we are!

* * *

I *Live in:*
Toronto, Canada.

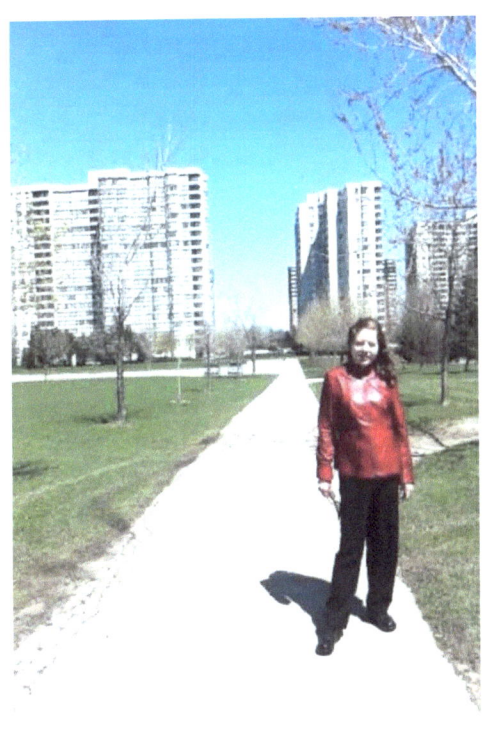

SHEILA BER, 2015.
(SHULLA)

This book is now available at:

www.amazon.com

www.createspace.com

www.kobobooks.com

www.indigo.chapters.ca